FUN WITH

FOOD

FACTS

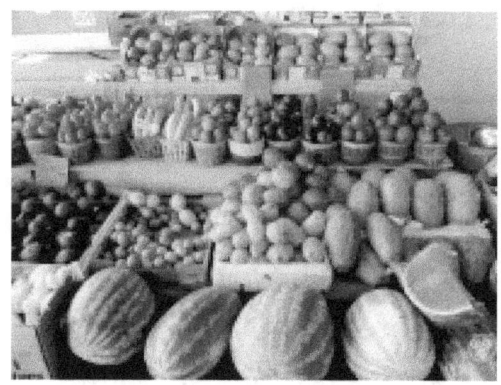

By Elizabeth K

This guide is to provide useful information to assist you in making your dietary choices, minus all the technical details you can't be bothered about. So leave that to the people who get obsessed about that sort of thing.

Table of Contents

Chapter One: FRUITS & VEGETABLES

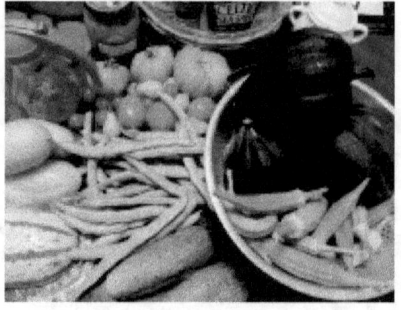

Vegetables are naturally low in fat and calories - but you already know that! That's why you don't like them! You want fat and calories, let's face it! Fat and calories are just so much fun and good-tasting. And even better looking! Nobody eats vegetables for dessert, do they? Fat and calories are the equivalent of that person you want to date!

Have you ever had a delicious item known as a Chinese donut? Yep, it's as awesome as it sounds. But the gooey center is of bean curd. Why? It's because bean curd supplies protein and tastes really good as a sweet paste. So in the Chinese diet you know how to combine the sweet with the healthy. How many fat Chinese people do you know, anyway? I bet not a one.

Besides the donut the Chinese also offer up a healthy but delicious alternative to an American banana split. Still using vanilla ice cream, instead of sugary sauces they finalize the dessert with fresh fruit.

The Chinese believe in developing real food and not sugary desserts. Needless to say, that is something you can easily do at home.

Big bowls of food do not produce a fat person. It's all in the balance of nutrition as well as the individual's metabolism, and there are certain things you can do to speed that up. Activity is one, and besides basic exercise try not to sit or be a couch potato for more than an hour at a time. When your body is sedentary so is the internal combustion engine.

VEGETABLES: are good for you. One reason is the lack of negative cholesterol. Cholesterol is a major negative in life. Cholesterol is one of those things that you have to monitor as you get older. That tells you how bad it is: life changing, as in life ending, when it's a big triple-digit number. How many people maneuver onto special diets and medications because of high cholesterol?

Many fruits and vegetables contain cancer inhibitors and the Big C is everyone's fear.

However, getting over that downer, let's get to wonderful stuff to eat.

FRUIT: is awesome! That is pretty much all you need to know. However one page does not make a book. It's not very informative either.

Fruit and vegetables can reduce your risk of certain cancers, of heart disease, of Type Two diabetes. So what's not to like? Specifically fruits and vegetables contain iron, fiber, folic acid, vitamins A & C. as well as potassium. They can also speed up your metabolism, if dieting is your concern.

Potassium helps you maintain a healthy blood pressure. Bananas and potatoes are a high source of potassium, but you don't want to overdue that. You might spike your potassium number, and too high a

count can lead to a heart issue you
don't want to have.

By the way, meaning you can eat a
potato or a banana for potassium
doesn't mean overdosing on
banana splits – not even the fresh
fruit variety - or potato chips or
French fries. I mean, that's like
saying fries or chips are real food,
and we know better, don't we?
You see, I knew you were heading
in that direction so I had to smack
you back to reality.

Fruit important to digest on as
regular a basis as possible are
apricots and peaches and especially
prunes.   But we don't want to hear
about sickeningly sweet prunes, so
forget about that for the moment.

If you watch any TV you know fiber
is an essential for reducing
constipation or its opposing
dynamic - diarrhea.

Fiber keeps you "regular" as the TV ads like to put it. It can also help those watching their weight, however, as foods with a heavy dose of fiber, such as beans and bananas, also fill you up as a diner, and consequently you eat less. And I know you're worried about that certain gaseous problem associated with beans consumption but it's not as bad as you think, because as your body becomes accustomed to beans as a supplement, that gaseous side effect goes away.

If you don't know about folic acid it assists the body in forming red blood cells. Pregnant women take folic acid to prevent some birth defects. Cardiologists are likely to prescribe folic acid to their cardiac patients. That single source proves an odd combination preventative. Just think about a pregnant woman who has a heart problem! You can bet she's on folic acid. Folic acid can be found in oranges, but I saw a cardiologist say it takes about 50 oranges a day to compensate for some recommended dosages and who wants to do that? It's not even advisable.

The most important thing about fruit is to eat the pulp, and not drink juice – not even prune juice, and I thought I wouldn't have to mention prunes again. Eating fruit in its whole form is especially important for diabetics, as juice tends to run through the system too rapidly, it is not a complex carbohydrate the way it is in its whole form.

Juice, even the natural variety – not artificially sweetened – runs through the system too quickly, does not require the longer lasting effect on the body as breaking down real food in the digestion process. So never buy or make juice when you have the option of eating whole fruit.

If you do have to buy juice, remember to check the juice content. Unless it is 100% juice – and the juice you want, not some other additive – don't even consider it as it has a filler of water and sugar. Not unless you are using juice as a substitute for a soda, in which case you might find yourself putting on weight you wouldn't have done with the soda. Yes, juice can make you fat! It often has higher calories than soda. And because it is JUICE you think to yourself it is healthy and you drink more and more of it, probably wondering why you are putting on weight as you are eating so healthy! Don't forget the more juice you are drinking and the higher calories, the more your diet is easing you into diabetes.

Another aspect to eating whole
fruit including the pulp is you are
doing something good for your
body instead of something bad.
And you already liked the flavor of
the fruit anyway; otherwise you
wouldn't have been buying the
juice.

If you think veggie juice is different,
think again. It's the same process.
Vegetables are also carbohydrates,
but good carbohydrates. Get rid of
the juice and eat the veggie,
reduced down if you have a food
processor that allows for that. You
want the integrity of the vegetable,
whole.

Calories are calories, and fruits and
vegetables generally lack protein to
balance it all out, so even if your
body is burning the calories, you
might be inching closer to diabetes

and you'll eventually receive a bad wake-up call from your physician.

If you've ever had a sugar rush from imbibing too much sweets or carbohydrates, one way to fix the problem quickly is to get up and start running in place until the nausea goes away. Or you can do a speed walk on a break, calisthenics, anything, to burn off the sugar. If you've had a real sugary dessert and side of sweet coffee, or a breakfast that was all carbs, that nausea may hit you rapidly. Do not wait it out, just take immediate physical action. It's an easy fix but surprisingly most people don't use it.

You best way of enjoying vegetables is to fry them or eat them in a salad.

Yes, you can fry food; you only have to minimize your oil and the choice of that oil. Olive oil and coconut oil are two of the recommended oils. They are known as healthy fats.

So it's not that bad! It's not like steamed veggies and flavorless food is your dreary future. You are not at the point of a macrobiotic diet (highly recommended as pure nutrition for cancer patients).

Naturally, the wonderful <u>avocado</u> is great in salads. But it's also great as a blended drink, or in a taco, or in a sandwich, or in an omelet, or as a dip, or anywhere except a soup. A warm avocado is not the recommended way to serve it, but I've heard tell you can fry them too.

The proper avocado is ripe when firm but slightly soft and the texture on your tongue is like that of butter. Now if you don't like avocados you are probably not from California, Mexico or South America. And if you are from these locales and you still hate avocados, you should move. An avocado is basically the official fruit of all these regions. Oh, yes, an avocado is a fruit. The short way of realizing a fruit, when in doubt, is they have pits. Either it's really small seeds, like in an orange or a large pit in the center of the fruit, like you'll find in a pear, an apple, or an avocado.

Another fruit that may surprise you is the tomato. Most cultures treat a tomato the same as an avocado, as an all-purpose fruit, except the tomato is one step up, as it also can be utilized better in a variety of sauces and hot meals. But you probably grew up eating spaghetti with marinara sauce and already know this. What you may not know is the type of acid the tomato contains makes it not great for certain digestive disorders, especially acid reflux. If you have GERT, it is advisable you resist consuming a tomato in any form. You'll find your side-effects much diminished.

Coffee and tea also contain an unhealthy acid content for GERT sufferers.

Apricots are your super-food if you're a smoker as it helps prevent lung cancer.

Asparagus is great for the kidneys.

Beets are fantastic for dieters, as it assists in flushing out fat.

Broccoli has fantastic iron, especially important and well-known to vegetarians or people with chronic anemia.

Cabbage stimulates the immune system as well as other things.

Carrots are great fighting cholesterol and preventing constipation.

Celery assists patients with arthritis as it contains Vitamin A.

Citrus Fruits in general fight viruses, since they contain Vitamin C.

Cranberries can prevent kidney stones. If you do have kidney stones, cranberries won't cure it.

Figs could be considered another superfood. Along with Prunes, they are a natural laxative and they aid in digestion. Oddly, figs can eliminate roundworms, perhaps due to being a laxative.

Garlic stimulates the immune system and relieves congestive issues like bronchitis. So for those winter cough sufferers, add on the garlic.

Grapes help prevent osteoporosis.

Horseradish relieves the sinuses which is great during weed and pollen season.

Lemons are a great acid trip! They may block cancer, and – as we know from history related to those long sea voyages - prevents scurvy. And you can't have lemonade without lemons anyway. Or have lemon with tea (iced or hot). Lemons also go great with fish and seafood. Lemon juice can be squeezed into a salad or pasta dish. You can see there's been a development in how to incorporate lemons in every dietary way possible, probably because of the long-ago fear of scurvy.

Lettuce, the basic iceberg variety, is roughage to help flush out the body. If you're having a salad, you should have it in a combination of greens for the most beneficial effect, such as adding spinach and romaine. This will also add flavor to your salad.

Onions and Pears help lower cholesterol.

Pineapples, Radishes and Sauerkraut flush fat from the body.

Soybeans have lecithin and lecithin inhibits the absorption of fat. In this way it works to prevent gallstones.

Tomatoes prevent appendicitis.

Peppers have a variety of uses – in hot or cold meals like salads or sandwiches - and they should be a part of every diet. If you ever have too much of a good thing and are reaching for that glass of water, the water won't help. What will help is dairy, so make it a glass of milk and the burn will reduce. (Dairy as an occasional thing, of course, an emergency standby.)

A way to add flavor to your salad or any meal is by eating your food at room temperature instead of too cold, as the freeze on the food inhibits flavors. The same with food that is too hot in temperature, as well.

If you need a cheese topping for this wonderful salad you're putting together, make it parmesan. You can sprinkle a bit and maximize the flavor of this pungent cheese without using more than your fat and cholesterol level can tolerate. If you're a popcorn aficionado replacing butter with sprinkled parmesan is healthier and still flavorful.

Your major issue – let's face it – when putting together a salad is the amount of cleaning, cutting and dicing you have to do with all the greenery. You probably think a salad takes too long, and you're right. So try to make it an enjoyable part of your day. Get all Zen over it. If you're on your own, watch a cooking show on TV for some motivation or listen to the news so you can maximize your time and enjoy a dual-focus. You'll start feeling proud of yourself. You'll start to fancy yourself a gourmet or even a career as a private chef. But don't take your eyes off the prize – the cut veggies – while you are chopping away. You don't want an accident and even the best chefs in the world experience a cut now and then.

Here's the secret – the more you do stuff like this, the more you enjoy the process. You will get to the point you are so domestic in the kitchen you imagine you are just as knowledgeable as all those chefs on TV. You'll be starting off with the easy vegetables, the ones you are already familiar with, but after a while you'll gain in confidence and start branching out, no pun intended. You'll try new mixes of vegetables and probably start making your own salad dressing as well, perhaps even giving bottles of the stuff away as gifts. Once more you will be fancying yourself with a new career. All this effort will do loads for your confidence in the kitchen.

If your specialty is peppers, you'll start bottling your own brand of hot sauce.

Overall, though, try and be careful in regards the dressings you choose, because you need to look at the calorie and fat from calories and make some good decisions. It's not just trans-fat you should avoid like the plague.

What you can do is start off using your normal grandiose helping of dressing and then gradually reduce the amount of dressing until you have a standard size salad with only a fraction of the dressing you used to use: especially if your salads tended to resemble a soup back when you started. You might get down to just a spoonful of dressing. This, of course, is if you're using a store bought unhealthy dressing rather than a healthier alternative at home.

Remember just because it looks good and says it is healthy, it may not be. You are responsible for your store-bought choices.

This is where that sprinkling of parmesan cheese comes in handy. But eventually work towards eliminating all cheese, except for special occasions, and a special occasion does not mean anytime your favorite TV show is on.

Another way to reduce dressing, and speed up your metabolism as well, is to add spice, something with a punch to it, such as <u>cayenne</u>, or start adding <u>onions</u> and <u>peppers</u>, even some jalapenos. <u>Jalapenos</u> have a flavor to match their knockout punch. Certain spices wake up your palate but also your metabolism.

Remember how vampires loathe <u>garlic</u>? Well, you'd best get to like it as it has beneficial results for your stomach. But don't eat too much garlic or you will simply reek of it, which is probably why sensitive vampires are repulsed.

Remember the best thing about fruits and vegetables is they can be enjoyed raw, and that includes the makeup of any fruit or veggie salad. Reducing cooking reduces mistakes made in the kitchen.

As you start exploring your choices you can add new ingredients and variants so you're not having the same thing every day.

And remember to add nuts to any veggie or fruit salad, as nuts such as walnuts and almonds will provide the healthy variety of fat and protein your body requires. A healthy diet does not mean eliminating all fat from the diet.

Mixing your greens is great. You shouldn't have just one leafy

vegetable in your salad, but two or
three varieties, as mentioned. But
also add cabbage of any type, as
you can mix it up and the greens
add flavor all their own, now
combined with the cabbage which
adds a spicy accent.

The wonder food of the ages is
beans. I can never talk enough
about beans! Beans are the secret
to longevity and don't doubt it.

A bland flavor on their own, just
like the protein tofu, the advantage
to that is they can be mixed into
just about anything, soup or salad,
you can even have it on the side of
an omelet. Or do scrambled eggs
with the beans included, maybe
adding some spices to increase the
flavor. Or mash it up and put it in a
sandwich as an additional spread.
The advantage to bland tofu and
beans is they absorb the flavors in

the ingredients surrounding them. If you can find it, some tofu varieties are pre-packed with flavor so it's already to taste.

If you're doing health-food drinks beans and tofu can be dropped into that blender just as well as anything else.

It's not a bad thing to plan out your meals every day and already have decided how you're going to incorporate those items.

If you're worried about cooking beans from its raw state, don't be. It's not that intimidating. What you can do is put a portion that will last you about a week – maybe 1 lb. for a single person – into a pot and put water over it. Let the beans sit in water for hours before heating the water to a boil and then taking it off the boil. This is the process for cooking beans. You may have to do that up to three times before the beans are soft enough to be soft. But that's all it takes. Drain the beans and you've got your supply.

Spinach has a different flavor when it's cooked vs raw. Most people enjoy raw spinach but have a problem with the odd flavor induced when it is cooked. But the warm spinach salad is very popular and certainly spinach in the raw is popular in a basic salad. Another way you can take advantage of iron heavy spinach is if you keep that kettle of soup going, because just as you were adding beans (protein; iron; calcium; vitamins A, B & C; etc.) to your soup, you can also drop in the spinach leaves.

Spinach is a miracle vegetable. If you have access to a garden, you should be planting spinach so you're able to utilize it.

Raw <u>cauliflower</u> and <u>broccoli</u> are great in salads. Some people use these veggies as finger food, alongside a dip, but if you're dieting or watching your fat content that's not advisable. Dips are extremely fattening.

Try frying <u>Brussel Sprouts</u> if you've never liked them before. You'll find you've changed your mind. Fry in coconut oil or olive oil and add spice.

The freshest ingredients are the healthiest. Think in terms of deterioration/corruption upon the death of something, the same thing happens to fruits and vegetables once they are picked. They are slowly dying from that point onward, so already one day after you have picked a vegetable or fruit, it's already one day less nutrient rich than the day before.

By the time produce shows up in the store shelves it is already days later. Just think of it this way: if you were buying fish off the boat at a dock, would you be choosing the fish they caught days ago, or the one they caught today?   Flash freezing stops the corruption process. But how much in the produce section of the grocery store or produce stand is flash frozen? It is a weird thought but sometimes the frozen produce section in the store has the freshest items. Just look for flash frozen.

To stick to a healthy eating pattern, planning out your grocery list and your meals in advance is a must. Otherwise you're likely to give into impulse and order that pizza or drive through that take-out window!

Not that you can't do that now and then. It's a good idea to shake up your body's expectations, to prevent your metabolism from becoming too complacent. Some people call it a cheat day, like day seven is for indulging oneself. You can take advantage of that to satisfy cravings you had during the week. Guess what? You've scheduled your craving from Tuesday, let's say, only now you don't have that craving anymore. The important thing is you executed command over your body by not indulging yourself before it was allowed.

Veering back and forth in weight up to five pounds isn't anything critical, so don't sweat the small stuff. As you effectively confuse your body, there will be minor weight fluctuations.

Food With Food Facts   Elizabeth K

Remember what you've always
been told, never shop for food
when you're hungry, and best to go
after you've already eaten,
otherwise you'll buy stuff you
never needed nor intended.

Chapter Two: FATS

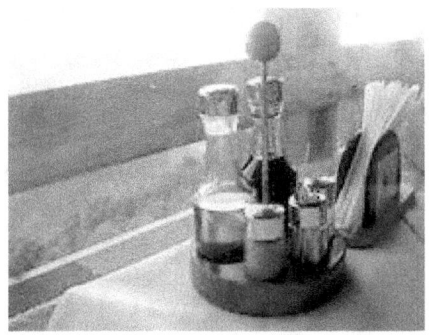

Yes, there are healthy fats. The most famous of these are olive oil and avocados, and even the healthy protein source – almonds. But it's the oils that are most famous for contributing healthy high saturated fats.

(Negative saturated fats are those associated with animal and animal by-products.)

Extra Virgin Olive Oil is used to lower blood pressure. It can also help prevent stroke and heart attacks. Italians like to dip their bread into olive oil and use olive oil as a staple in their pasta dishes.

Many people consider the Italians (and the Greeks) to be the best-looking people on the planet and what they have in common is their love of olive oil. Remember the olive tree was gifted to the Greeks by Athena and the gods never gave a better present to humankind.

The primary benefit of Coconut Oil is how great it is for diabetics and it assists in the digestion of calcium and magnesium. As an aside, it assists in healthy skin and hair.

Coconut oil is 90% saturated fat, and saturated fat is a bad thing. Saturated fats are meat by-products like dairy and palm and coconut oils. However these oils with saturated fats have been ingested for thousands of years before heart disease became a staple of human existence.

The really controversial elements in the progression of heart disease are polyunsaturated vegetable oils like corn, safflower and canola.

Did you know *margarine* was developed to have fatal consequences? It was created as a poison to feed to fowl. Coloring was added and that's how it became sold to humans as a – get this, supposedly, healthy! – substitute for butter. Let's face it, the mind boggles.

If you want a source other than fish for Omega-3, it is either thru a superfood you can purchase off the shelf, or <u>Flax Seed</u> oil. Currently there is <u>Flax Milk</u> on the dairy shelf so you can have it in place of milk with your cereal or coffee. As a supplement it requires no more than a tablespoon a day. More than that can have negative effects on the body.

<u>Hemp Oil</u> is loaded with multi-vitamins and minerals but also contains a 3-to-1 ratio of Omega-3 fatty acids to Omega-6 fatty acids. As well, the oil contains sitosterol, which lowers cholesterol and tocopherols which have antioxidant properties. It is loaded with anti-oxidants.

Hemp oil comes in another form, a solid, that some people swear is beneficial as it is rubbed on ailing parts of the body (injured or arthritic joints). Other people say it is a placebo, meaning the person using it has fooled themselves into thinking it has produced beneficial gains.

Chapter Three:
CARBOHYDRATES

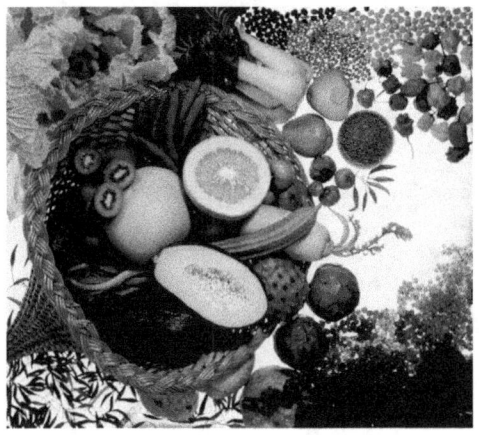

Carbohydrates are required to create glucose which is the body's fuel. So getting rid of carbs in a carb-free diet can be you're attempting a marathon but capable of no more than a sprint.

There are <u>simple carbohydrates</u> and <u>complex carbohydrates</u>.

Complex carbohydrates are desirable as they are foods that take longer to break down, usually high in fiber, like fresh fruit. Whole grains, beans and vegetables are the same as fruit, they are complex carbs.

Simple Carbs are fast fixes, sometimes known as a sugar high, usually to be found in soda, fruit juice and snack food.

If you are dieting you delete added sugar items such as *cookies*, *cakes*, *candies* and ice *cream* from your diet. (They all start with C, did you notice?)

That is, unless you're having a cheat meal or day where you allow yourself an indulgence, which is something you have to work out in advance. You don't want any guilt trip afterwards.

Actually it is a good idea to have a cheat day or meal, because this confuses the body about what is normal, what is to be anticipated and keeping your body somewhat off-guard is how you might avoid that plateau effect every dieter undergoes.

A major dessert component can be angel food cake, as it contains no fat, but it is hardly diet food.

Sugar in WHOLE fruit is natural and not to be eliminated for its own sake.

There is a debate whether diet drinks have the same effect upon the body as a sugar additive drink. So diet soda is as bad for you as regular soda? It could be. The body seems to treat sweeteners all the same.

Breads are largely to be eliminated by dieters, they are bad carbohydrates. The odd thing is a study has shown the sourdough variety takes the longest to break through the body, over that of grain-variety, so if you have to eat bread, sourdough is the healthier alternative.

The sandwich known as a wrap was developed to provide people with sandwich alternatives that did not include bread.

Chapter Four:
PROTEINS

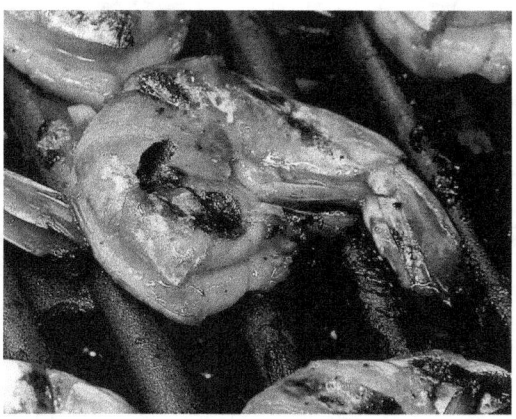

Proteins can be controversial because there is a silent battle of wills between vegetarians and meat-eaters. But don't worry; we're not going to have that war here.

To clarify, proteins are components of all living cells and include enzymes, hormones, and antibodies. That's very scientific, I know, but I had to put it in here somewhere.

Proteins are made up of amino acids, which our bodies, in the main, automatically manufacture.

Finding proteins to eat are easy as they come in all the food groups, from dairy products including cheeses (the harder the cheese the greater the protein content) and yogurts (the Greek variety is preferable), to meats, fish, and nuts. And don't forget beans, including soy and tofu (which, by itself, has a long range of products to offer).

Most people – especially chefs – use the word protein to describe the star of their dish, the meat or fish or seafood product on the plate. The other elements, the so-called starch and vegetables, are placed on the plate in order to produce a well-rounded meal, so these other items service the protein.

Did you know the U.S. (famous) food pyramid has now reduced the status of protein? It is lower now in stature, as the health risks associated with meat and even the daily amount of fish you can consume, have become well-researched. Protein is not as important as it was once assumed to be, at least not in as high an amount as previously considered.

But protein is vital, only in smaller doses than previously thought; as well the type of protein consumed is the most important part of the equation.

It has also been discerned the average American – very focused on meat products as part of any everyday meal – ingests far more protein than the body requires, in fact each day they may consume three to five days' worth of their body's protein needs.

Even worse, often dieters reduce or eliminate the amount of carbohydrates they consume in favor of an all-protein diet. That may work in the short-term, but how likely are they to keep the weight off? Especially as the body becomes weighted down with the protein, the metabolism stops functioning properly, and you have no energy left. You probably don't sleep well either. So what have you gained? The loss of some poundage but that's probably temporary and you're really not feeling good either. Certainly your body is not enthused by any all-protein diet. You are facing both short-term and long-term health risks.

Animal products and by-products inhibit your metabolism and are related to all sorts of illnesses, especially cancer and heart disease.

When you're twenty years old,
you're not thinking about this. But
often how you eat affects your
body ten years down the line, and
that is especially true for chronic or
fatal complications to develop.

Pork is an iffy proposition. It is
likely the reason for pork being a
forbidden food to the ancient
Hebrews is because when it's not
cooked properly, pork begets
worms, which can be lethal if not
treated right away (the worms can
travel from your intestines into
your brain). Pork does not have to
be overcooked, to the point of
being well-done, but it definitely
needs to be cooked properly for
consumption.

So: you are what you eat. Did you
want to be a cow?

Did you know cheese – extremely
delicious on its own - is the hardest
substance for the body to digest?
Well, now you do. Of course it's a

cause of high cholesterol numbers.
The more cheese you eat, the
higher your cholesterol needle is
going to move. It's extremely high
negative numbers on the
cholesterol scale.

If you need to reduce cholesterol,
immediately decrease or eliminate
cheese from your diet. Guess
what? You'll also be losing weight.

A cow produces milk for her baby
in order for the baby to swiftly
progress into a few hundred
pounds behemoth. So think of that
in relation to your own body,
replacing your small self with that
of the nearest cow.

Did you also consider that humans
are the only species routinely
ingesting the milk of another
species into their diet? And cheese
comes from milk, we all know that.
Being raised on milk, we take it for
granted this is normal, so we never
bother to think about it. But it is

COW or GOAT or some other type of milk. Frankly, it should freak you out. Then again, it is delicious, and an accepted society norm, so I forgive you.

But most people grow intolerant to milk as they age. The sensitivity comes from the fermentation. The bloating and gas and even the sharp pains from the gastrointestinal area are a result.

Fish is a great source of protein. It is a super-food. It has so many health benefits it would make you think fish should be consumed all day with every meal. It works against some cancers, against arthritis, and heart attacks and asthma. It also aids in mental energy and inhibits blood clots.

Fish is great. But some fish are fattier than others. And fish shouldn't be consumed every day. Also take into consideration the health of the waters in which the catch was caught. Many times the areas have been polluted and the product is unattainable. Don't fry the fish unless you can leave it to its natural state when cooking, which means no added ingredients. Let the flavor of the fish come out; don't bog it down with sauces or butter.

Butter is not your friend. But if you settle on one of those all-things-go days once a week, or for a dining out meal, then by all means allow yourself some indulgence. Call it the indulgence day or meal.

A breakfast staple is eggs. Many people have intolerance to eggs, specifically the yolk. The yolk is fat. The whites are protein. As stated previously, never consume raw eggs.

The sources of proteins that have staying power and are consumed in cultures where weight and longevity don't seem to be an issue are <u>beans</u>, which is nature's superfood. In fact, fish and beans are often a staple of these cultures.

There are by-products of beans, which are <u>soy</u> and <u>tofu</u>. There are also vegetarian versions of salami, bologna and turkey that are made from gluten or soy. They replicate the look and flavor of the meat they are meant to replace, for those vegetarians wanting a greater variety of food in their diet. Vegetarians were largely raised with meat as a staple, too, remember?

Nuts of all varieties contain protein, and the best snacking food is raw <u>almonds</u>. You can live on a diet of almonds and <u>apples</u> as a great way to manage your weight. Apples are another superfood! Never be hungry as you pretty much snack all day. Between those two items you have a healthy diet going for you. It may not be exciting, but it will work.

Chapter Five:
SUPERFOODS

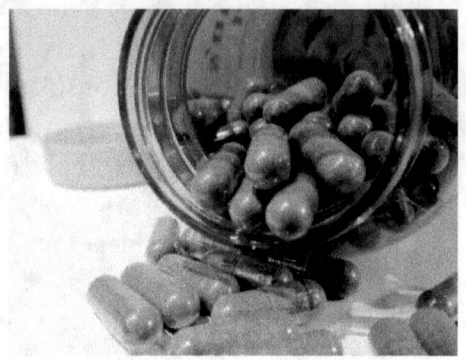

There is so much controversy regarding supplements and vitamins that you literally make a choice in what you believe. But the main thing to do is to feed your body, which means you have to know its needs. That is going to be based upon your age and state of health and your fitness level.

Are you an active person or a passive person? If you are a

passive person, ask yourself why? Are you ashamed to work out in public? Many heavyweight people are. But no matter the cause of your inhibition, there are plenty of exercises you can do in the privacy of your home, for instance riding an exercise bike. The trick is to find a comfortable seat cushion on the bike, so you are not flinching the entire time you're riding it. Also schedule a firm time every day to get onto that bike, maybe during your favorite half-hour show.

So the question is, if there's not a physical disability then why aren't you more active? Even if you're healthy, start slowly, by taking a walk, or do something that can increase your social network, such as taking a Tai Chi class.

Did you know Tai Chi is great for the energy level of the body? That is where the Chi comes in. Did you know cardiac patients see an improvement in their state of health once they commence a Tai Chi regimen? Cardiologists often recommend a Tai Chi regimen to their patients. The maneuvers look so basic, because it's not an impact sport. But who says an impact sport is great for the body? Actually it's just the opposite. Bruising force amounts to a bruising. Force equals impact and something's got to give, and that means a stress or an injury to some part of your person.

Low impact, aerobic, exercise is the best activity for improving your balance and maintaining body tone. Naturally that means yoga, swimming, dancing. Yep, go dancing! Dancing is exercise, really fun but exhausting exercise. The old rules apply; don't over-extend yourself in any activity you undertake. Don't think you're having fun and then suddenly you're going into cardiac arrest.

Are you having aches and pains or digestive disorders? Then exercise isn't your main issue.

Even if you share the same sex, age and weight and activity level of the person standing next to you, it could be you have different supplemental needs. Did you know the famous BMI (body mass index) is totally ridiculous? It is because it only counts a person's weight and height, not taking into account the individual's state of health, let alone the build as in small, medium or large.

Doctors love to prescribe pills. Some of those pills may be heavy in side effects.

Regarding supplements many people blend the pills into their smoothies. (Just remember to never, ever use a raw egg in a smoothie. Raw eggs are unhealthy to eat. Never feed an egg to a pet. It is a common source of dogs with a chronic itch.) Though supplements probably are more easily absorbed when it's consumed in a beverage, that doesn't mean your body requires all the supplements you are taking.

And supplements are expensive, right? So why buy something you don't need? Is it for peace of mind? A "better take this in case I need it" affect? Then you've got a lot of spare cash, huh, and maybe a personal chef as well?   And what about ingesting something your body doesn't need? Could you be causing another side effect?

There is a school of thought no supplements should be required when you have a healthy diet. But most people think that's pushing your luck.

In order to learn if you have any pressing or tentative health risk, you should obtain a screening, which will be part of a general blood work.

When it comes to OTC ("over the counter") supplements, you need to obtain the best brands. You need to have faith what you are paying for is what you are getting.

Did you know some store brands got in trouble for labeling their supplements one way while the contents were something else? It happened quite a bit with people buying gingko biloba and getting horseweed in place of it. So fraud is rampant in an industry where nutritional supplements are not under the province of the Food and Drug Administration (USA). (Only prescriptions medications have to have FDA approval before being marketed and made available to the general public.) But the outright fraud is what got those store brands in trouble, if they'd been selling the product advertised on the label that would have been okay – whether the supplement works as recommended, well, that's buyer beware. All nutrient and dosage recommendations are per the manufacturer label and unreliable as well.

As you get older you are more likely to need prescriptions and supplements to stay in as good shape as possible. Certainly essentials like calcium are an increased need that diet alone can't meet. And it's a delicate balance, as the fragility of bones is prevalent but too much calcium can make your bones too brittle.

There are Amino Acids the body doesn't manufacture on its own and it's good to know where it can be found naturally. Otherwise look for it as a (reliable) supplement you can purchase:

ISOLEUCINE & LEUCINE: These provide muscle fuel and can be found naturally in meat byproducts and seeds.

LYSINE: Is required for intestinal absorption of calcium and is necessary for collagen formation as well as helps produce antibodies.

METHIONINE: Helps the liver metabolize fats and assists in collagen formation.

PHENYLALANINE: This is important in producing brain chemicals and converts to Tyrosine which in turn manufactures Epinephrine, Norepinephrine and Thyroid hormones.

THREONINE: Helps the body in stabilizing blood sugar and is necessary for the formation of tooth enamel, collagen and elastin. (A supplement that also assists in blood sugar processing is cinnamon, which is great because it can be added to many things, including smoothies, tea and coffee beverages. Cinnamon is a great spice that is a superior supplement and one people love and that's a rare thing.)

TYPTOPHAN: Produces Serotonin, a brain chemical (notoriously) involved in mood regulation.

<u>VALINE</u>: Promotes growth, tissue repair and blood sugar regulation.

Many of your store supplements might be branded in a superfood category all its own, including one pound package containers or in pill form. When you look at the label information pay attention to what they say this particular form of superfood is supposed to be containing.

For instance, if you buy a superfood in powder form, you can add it to any liquid including water – usually a single teaspoon – and that promises much better absorption than any pill. And you can add a powder supplement to any liquid you drink, including the infamous smoothie.

There are already substances that are heavy in omegas and B-12 or various vitamins and minerals, so you can eliminate separate purchases of those items when you are getting those substances in another form. There's no reason to double-up on any OTC nutritional supplement.

Often one supplement you are searching for is already inclusive in another product, so once you get your needs organized you can start minimizing your expenditures.

For superfoods to munch on, consider apricots, walnuts, almonds, apples, avocados, cashews. If you're munching on nuts, make sure they are in the raw state. To have added flavoring or salt means your superfood is not-so-super anymore.

When frying your meal, consider coconut oil, vegetarian oil, peanut oil and the famous olive oil. Not for nothing did Athena present the Greeks with the olive tree.

For breakfast, consider oatmeal, the slow cooking variety. Add a low calorie or natural maple syrup to it for sweetening. Instead of a dairy milk or cream, use a coconut milk or almond milk (you know these are not real milk-based, right?). They come in regular and unsweetened so you have a choice. If you have a low tolerance for sweet foods, this is a good thing as you will look for ways to reduce your caloric intake.

Apple cider vinegar is often added to salads and soups. Some people take a tablespoon of it in water, daily. That makes a lot of people gag. However it is great for cleansing the body of toxins, and works especially well in aiding

digestion and easing arthritis
(flushing out toxins).

Remember, fish is preferable over
meat. White meat is preferable
over red meat. That's a mantra.